Intermitte

The 30-Day Schedule to Reversing Anxiety, Regaining Energy and Maximizing Productivity

Table of Contents

Introduction

I want to thank you and congratulate you for downloading my book ***Intermittent Fasting: The 30-Day Schedule To Reversing Anxiety, Regaining Energy and Maximizing Productivity***.

This book contains proven steps and strategies on how to practice the Palaeolithic art of intermittent fasting (IF).

The approach taken is to first look at the theory behind IF, then to address the benefits of a dietary approach to management of ailments and maximization of wellbeing in general, before moving onto the specific benefits of our ***30-Day Schedule to Reversing Anxiety, Regaining Energy, and Maximizing Productivity***.

Along the way we will outline a foundation of scientific research and literature on the method, and assess what the method can do for you, whatever your age, lifestyle and specific requirements.

Thanks again for downloading this book, I hope you enjoy it!

Chapter 1: Food and Medication Overload and the Dietary Approach

Dieting is the conscious control of what food we humans consume. In the course of our history, dieting is a relatively new phenomenon. Indeed for most of it, our diet was controlled by availability - when Stone Age man managed to kill the wooly mammoth he ate well, when he didn't, he went hungry.

The first texts on dieting can be traced to 18th century England and the practice became widespread in that country in the Victorian era, with the first popular diet being named after the corpulent undertaker George Banting. This consisted of four square meals per day including meats, greens, fruit and wine (not the biggest sacrifice you may say, and possibly why Banting's book remains in print to this day).

When the Stone Age man first hunted the mammoth, he used sticks and with these alone didn't have a great success - each hunt could result in a number of human deaths. So he used our innate creativity to invent a flint-bladed spear, and the success rate improved, but it was still a dangerous enterprise with more empty seats at the dinner table each time.

Then one day a bright member of the tribe suggested hunting HERDS of mammoths over a steep drop, leading them to plummeted to the bottom. This revolutionary step forward brought much rejoicing;

until it was realized that all of the region's mammoths had been wiped out in short order, and only a fraction of what had been killed could even be eaten in enough time before the rest was spoiled.

That is a classic *PROGRESS TRAP*, and we mention it here because it is precisely what humanity has gotten itself into when it comes to diet and human health. Particularly in the West, but increasingly globally as middle-class incomes and lifestyles improve - we just need to look at the chronic diseases that have GROWN in frequency despite the stratospheric advances in medicine over the past century to know that something is amiss.

Diabetes, many forms of cancer, heart disease, sclerosis of the liver, even obesity as a discrete disease; these are a product of increasingly poor diet and sedentary lifestyles. And it's not only physical ailments: as we focus on here, mental health issues and anxiety have increased EXPONENTIALLY, yes because of greater awareness and the increasingly fast pace and complexity of life, but also because of our sedentary lifestyles and unhealthy diets.

A favorite statistic of mine is the fact that each day in the USA the food and drinks industries sell enough produce to supply every single person with almost 4000 calories – TWICE what is required. When we think about how much of that is in unhealthy, sugar, salt and fat laden fast food, ready meals, processed meats and sauces, confectionary, alcoholic products and - possibly most of all – soft drinks, we can see a truly frightening picture emerging.

Add in the dependence on the automobile that has been literally embedded in our environment through suburbanization; mechanization leading to a laying off people whose occupations require physical labor; and the ever-increasing time we spend in front of our myriad of devices with glowing screens; and a truly frightening healthcare picture emerges.

Unfortunately, modern humanity's answer to this global pandemic has been to medicate, medicate, MEDICATE. The culture of a pill for every ill, led by Big Pharma and its lobbyists and endorsed by a supplicant medical profession, leads to the treatment (with varying degrees of success) of *symptoms but not underlying causes.*

Say you have been to the doctor and diagnosed with type-2 diabetes following a blood-sugar test. You will most likely be placed on a glipizide- or glyburide-type medication to bring your levels down fast. Once this is achieved, however, the drugs will not get to the root of what caused your illness in the first place, and in many cases, neither will your physician.

This widespread approach is akin to dealing with a leaky roof by placing a bucket under a leaky roof, and once that bucket is nearly full replacing it with another bucket, then continuing to do this year after year, rather than replacing the faulty tile. To replace the tile, we need a more root-and-branch approach, which looks at overall health (physical and mental), health and wellbeing – that what makes us not only healthy but productive, happy and motivated humans.

Chinese medicine and other 'alternative' approaches have long advocated this method but it has only been in recent decades that the centuries-old practice of dieting and the concept of a HOLISTIC approach to wellbeing rather than the point-and-click approach of pharmacological medicine have begun to converge and gain traction in Western medicine.

Accordingly, there are a myriad of approaches each advocating a different diet for both general and specific health conditions. Whether it is the DASH diet for hypertension (**D**ietary **A**pproache**S** for **H**ypertension), the Atkins diet to burn fat, the Paleo (or caveman) diet which allows only foods that can be hunted or fished and reduces diabetes and heart conditions, there will be a sea of literature and a host of devotees and often equally vociferous doubters.

We do not have the space in this e-book to examine the pros and cons of all the leading diets, as we have studying the one in particular – 30-Day Intermittent Fasting – that I believe, from my studies and personal experience, that is the most effective and that offers the most rapid means (the fastest route one could say) to reducing anxiety, regaining lost energy and maximizing productivity.

So, without further ado let's jump right into it.

Chapter 2: Intermittent Fasting – What is it and how does it work?

2.1 Background

Intermittent fasting, or IF as we will refer to it from here on in, refers to any eating pattern that alternates between periods of fasting and periods of eating. Purists would say that it is therefore not a diet (it doesn't change *what* you eat only *when* you eat), though using our broad-based definition of diet as control of consumption we would say that it is. Besides, no matter what the approach adopted, people generally want the same outcomes from conscious control of their food intake and so it is more useful to put all in the one low-calorie pot.

It can be said that IF has been with us from the BEGINNING of life on earth. For away from the world of modern human civilization where we and our domesticated animals eat as and when we want to or are directed to, the norm for hundreds of millions of years has been to eat when food was AVAILABLE. This was the case for our Stone Age friends (one final mention for them), and has been and is the case for all wild fauna on earth to this day.

2.2 The Science Bit

Think of the python that has just engorged itself on the antelope to get a better understanding of IF – just like in all those Sunday evening wildlife shows on television.

As it swallows and ultimately digests and absorbs the antelope, the python is very much in the *fed state*. In the snake's case, it will be in this state for a week or so; for a human eating a normal meal it will typically be a period of around four hours from the time of taking the first bite.

In the fed state, insulin levels are high and the body burns very little fat, so sugar is stored in the liver which only has limited room and so starts to turn this excess sugar into more fat.

This process is called De-Novo Lipogenesis (which sounds like an up market and high-sugar producing Italian restaurant but literally means *making fat from new*). Some of this new *novo lipo* (new fat, technically glycogen) is stored in the liver, but as we know the liver has a storage limit and plenty to be getting on with anyway, so it pumps out the majority to the rest of body where there is literally no storage limit (think Henry VIII or Jabba the Hut), and it is this process that quite literally allows us to GET FAT via excessive sugar intake.

Following from this the body enters the *post-absorptive state* - which simply means that the body is no longer processing a meal. Post absorption for a human typically lasts a further four hours, which is eight hours in total after the meal, after which the body will enter the *fasted state* (our reptilian friend won't be getting to here for a good month or so).

In the fasted state, insulin levels are low and so it much easier for the body to burn off fat that has been inaccessible to it in the fed state. The body starts by burning off any accessible glycogen by breaking it down to glucose molecules as an energy source and only when that supply is exhausted that it moves to the body fat stored elsewhere – the process of weight loss.

2.3   Application

As you'll have figured out what this means is that in a typical day the body is likely to be only in the fasted state for a short period before breakfast, as we'll probably have at least three square meals through the day and a few snacks and drinks in between. If we stop and think about the word "breakfast", we can see it is quite literally "break" and "fast", the meal that BREAKS the FASTING. This is a word that's been around in the English language for over five hundred years, so we get an indication of the practice has been engrained into human culture.

One of the key benefits of IF is that it forces the body into this high fat-burning state in a regular and controlled manner. Many scholars of the theory would say that it aligns our body clock with our evolutionary design and with the rest of life on earth (for it will be some years yet before the routine driven by the weekly supermarket shop and regular mealtimes is bred into our DNA).

Indeed, some recent thinking in medicine has begun to question the entire "three square meal plus snacks" approach. Dr. Mark Mattson, professor of Neuroscience at The Johns Hopkins University has said the following which is worth quoting in its entirety as it gets to the heart of the matters under discussion here:

Why is it that the normal diet is three meals a day plus snacks? It isn't that it's the healthiest eating pattern ... I think there is a lot of evidence to support that. There are a lot of pressures to have that eating pattern, there's a lot of money involved. The food industry — are they going to make money from skipping breakfast like I did today? No, they're going to lose money. If people fast, the food industry loses money. What about the pharmaceutical industries? What if people do some intermittent fasting, exercise periodically and are very healthy, is the pharmaceutical industry going to make any money on healthy people?

So, it's only relatively recently that some experts such as Dr. Mattson have begun to rebel against a dietary status-quo that has prevailed from the late 19th century. This orthodoxy has been driven by the Kellogg's, Kraft's and Coca Colas of this world and their sisters in Big Pharma as opposed to by logic or, perish the thought, the notion of what is ACTUALLY better for us consumers.

Read on to find out how you can benefit from IF and the 30-day schedule.

Chapter 3: Why 30 Days? Intervals and Alternatives

3.1 Eat Less Food

The title of this book begins with the words "30-Day Schedule", so no prizes for guessing that we advocate a monthly IF plan for MAXIMUM results. To explain why that is, it is necessary to start with some explanation of the importance of the periods of intermittence, and the underlying theory behind this.

We've learnt that the primary rationale behind IF is to maximize, indeed increase greatly, periods of high FAT-BURNING (in contrast to sugar burning) in the body. Quite simply, if we're not eating, then the body must burn off its own fat reserves to give us the energy we need to function; just as in the case of a hibernating bear or a blubbery whale.

Another glaringly obvious benefit is that, for any given time interval, fasting while consuming the same amount of food in non-fasting periods will result in lower calorific intake – less stuff going into the body will lead to weight loss in anyone with a previously stable weight profile. There is also significant research to show that, at least for mice, lower caloric intake is associated with longevity.

The American rocker Stephen Stills of Crosby, Stills and Nash fame once told an interviewer that he was on the "ELF diet". When pressed what this new acronym represented in the canon of West Coast dietary fads, Stills replied "Eat Less Food". And so, it is also apparent that the duration of the fasting period will dictate how much less food is eaten overall.

Let's look next at some of the common fasting periods that inform variants of IF, before explaining the 30-day approach in detail.

3.2   Common IF Types

- **Eat-Stop-Eat:** Once or twice a week, depending on the intensity of your plan, take a complete 24-hour break from dinner one day until dinner the next (i.e. Thursday evening to Friday evening). This is a more difficult diet as initially at least you are likely to suffer hunger pangs towards the end of day two. The key benefit is in the longer fast time: stepping back to our science we are getting well into the fasting phase with its attendant benefits on a regular basis. We will be using Eat Stop Eat as the basis of our 30-day plan.
- **The 16/8 method (or Leangains)**: Eat for 16, fast for 8 would be too easy, so it's the other way around. For example, eating only between noon and 8pm. *16/8* is probably the MOST COMMON type of IF, as it is easy to achieve, if you are already a breakfast-dodger. A 16/8 plan on this schedule will allow for 16 hours of fasting time daily, giving the body some time to burn off its excess fat (stay in *ketosis*). One

issue many people have with this method is that they find it difficult to maintain calorie intake with fewer meals – it's harder to eat fewer bigger portions – and so end up losing more weight than they bargained for. 16/8 was developed by Martin Berkhan at LeanGains.com; go there for more detailed info on the method.

- **The 5:2 Diet:** Rather than complete fasting, *5:2* directs that the follower eats only 500-600 calories on two days of the week (about 20% of normal for a man, 25% for a woman). Focusing more on calorie reduction than IF, 5:2 is a popular diet that's easy to adopt particularly if you are creative with your food intake on fast days – though you can never really fool the body when it comes to low calorie substitutes.

- **Alternate Day Fasting:** Does exactly what it says on the tin, you fast every other day. This is obviously quite an extreme diet to fit into your lifestyle, and many followers will follow a modified approach allowing 500 calories on fasting days (a 4:3 diet if you will).

- **The Warrior Diet:** As the name suggests not for the fainthearted, this diet, popularized by Ori Hofmekler, consists of fasting for most of the day then eating all your calories in one sitting at the end of the day. It's really a 20:4 split as opposed to 16:8 and is ideal for people whose routines and jobs regularly involve large dinners in social settings (wine is a great way of piling on the calories!). The advantage is in the longer fasting period which allows significant burning of body fat; the main difficulty is in working it into the daily routine for most of us - that and probably a lot of indigestion.

- **Skipped Meals:** To the other end of the scale from the Warrior Diet. Skipped Meals is just that; if you're hungry, eat, and if not then skip it until the next meal. You can follow a more planned regime (e.g. skip every teatime), or simply use it a means to overcome the routine of consuming food on the same daily schedule for no other reason than it's because it's what you do. A good introductory IF method, you can work this into your daily life as an evolutionary as opposed to revolutionary method.

3.3   The 30-Day Plan

From the above we can see various ways to take us on the same destination to a lower fat, higher energy lifestyle. Each mode of travel is different and some are undoubtedly faster and more unsettling than others, but all are based on the principles that we discussed above.

Our method advocates a 30-day plan, for the simple reason that 30 days is a short enough time window for most of us to retain enthusiasm and COMMITMENT to a new dietary schedule, and long enough to see and more importantly to feel the benefits that will convince us to make IF central to our lives long term.

The core plan proposed here is based around Eat-Stop-Eat, with fasting for two 24 hour days each week (supper to supper).

For the remainder of the time you should eat as normal, though before committing it's a good idea to take a step back and look at your own normal – if you are forever eating junk food on the go, or miss meals sporadically through the week, or generally do not have a balanced and consistent dietary intake, then it is strongly advisable to commit to remedying this before you undertake the trial.

Note: If you are pregnant, are diabetic, under eighteen years of age, underweight, on prescribed medications of any kind or generally in poor health then you should not

undertake the 30-day plan. If you have any doubts as to your suitability or fitness, please speak to your physician.

Other than this, the rules are simple:

- FAST between the allocated times twice a week, or eight to nine times through the period (preferably spaced as equidistant as your schedule allows), and wait to see the results.
- You should weigh yourself at the start, middle and end of the thirty days as a minimum and it's advisable and useful to take more periodic checks to see how your body responds to the intervals of fasting and eating. It is also interesting to monitor daily calorie intake (sparkpeople.com is one location where you can try out a free estimator) and plot some trends over the period – particularly if you intend to use the approach repeatedly, as we believe you will.

If two (2) fast days in every seven (7) seems too arduous given your circumstances, then benefits can be seen from a one day fast, or from one 24 hour fast and 18 hour fast. Tailor the method to your needs and requirements. Remember this is all for YOUR benefit - it's not a competition, and if you fall off the wagon and eat during a fast day, then just dust yourself down and get straight back on the horse. Yes, the benefits are maximized by following the schedule, but even if you don't do this religiously at your first attempt, THE

MORE YOU DO THE BETTER YOU WILL FEEL AND MORE PRODUCTIVE YOU WILL BE.

At the end of our challenge we will have reduced our calorie intake by approximately 30% if we follow the full plan. For the vast majority of us, this will be achieved with no detrimental impact on how we lead our lives days to day, but rather will provide clear and immediately benefits in terms of our mental health and anxiety, our energy levels and our productivity – we turn to these in detail below.

In addition, we will be re-programming ourselves, re-attuning to evolutionary and cultural basics of what it is to be human. At the cellular level, we will direct our cells to obtain most of our energy needs from the fatty deposits throughout our bodies as opposed to the glycogen in our livers. In doing so we will not only lose weight (though intensive weight loss is not our goal) and begin to optimize our body mass index (BMI), but we will free ourselves from constantly thinking about our next meal and learn to manage hunger pangs and take back control of our bodies.

Finally, we will be fighting back against the food conglomerates that bombard us with unnecessary product with their multi-billion-dollar advertising budgets, and the major pharmaceuticals whose arms they drive us into to seek unsatisfactory remedies for our self-inflicted ailments.

Chapter 4: The 30-Day Plan – Physical Health Benefits

"A little starvation can really do more for the average sick man than can the best medicines and the best doctors" - Mark Twain

In this section, we look in further detail at the clinically proven health benefits of the 30-day plan. In the next section, we will translate these to tangible benefits in reducing anxiety, restoring energy, and maximizing productivity.

We'll show that Mark Twain was right all those years ago, and that you can reap the benefits without starving yourself (Twain wasn't known for his sensitive use of language, this is the guy who once threatened to dig up Jane Austen and beat her back to death with her own shinbone).

4.1 Insulin, Glycogen and Fat Burning

As covered under the science, the primary benefit of IF and our 30-day plan for the vast majority will be the decreased period of INSULTION PRODUCTION in the body, driving a virtuous cycle of increased body fat burning.

In his bestselling IF text *Eat Stop Eat*, Brad Pilon showed that the amount of stored fat released for oxidation (burning) through the lipolysis process increased by over 50% after only 24 hours of fasting.

We'll be getting seven such hits in our 30 days, and the benefits will be dramatic.

4.2   Weight Loss

The first think everyone thinks of when anything to do with dieting is mentioned. Due to your decreased calorific intake (around 30% for our plan remember), your body will have the necessary conditions to not only stop weight gain, but also to lose weight. Research has shown that any time we fast for a significant period (>18 hours), we lose two to three pounds in weight.

How much you lose will depend upon a lot of factors, including your metabolic rate (which drives your normal weight gain/loss profile), current weight, your diet and how active you are. As you become familiar with the 30-day regime you will be able to monitor how it is impacting on your body and tweak your food intake and level of exercise to optimize it for you. As we've said, weight loss is not the primary objective for most people who subscribe to the plan, and, particularly if you are fit and healthy, it's possible to reap the benefits without losing a single pound and maintaining your muscle mass – more on that later.

4.3   Hormonal Benefits

As your body burns off more fat reserves several secondary processes are invoked or optimized which in turn derive additional benefits for us, particularly at the hormonal level.

4.4   Adrenaline

Adrenaline and noradrenalin (also known as epinephrine and norepinephrine) are the body's fight or flight hormones, i.e. in times of stress they increase the blood flow and the oxygen getting to the muscles, essentially increasing your capacity to deal with the situation by fighting or by running away. Physical symptoms are a thumping heart rate and sweating, and mental alertness and focus is increased. Mentally, ALERTNESS and FOCUS increases.

It has been shown that all IF programs serve to increase adrenaline levels, because the body is already in a heightened state of fat burning and not simply adding to its fat reserves. The benefits of this response in terms of energy and productivity levels are apparent, however care does need to be taken in controlling the levels released, which we will explore further below.

4.5   Growth Hormone

Human Growth Hormone (HGH) is produced the pituitary gland, not only for children (for whom it is essential), but in all of us. HGH is then released into the bloodstream, only momentarily, before it is sent to the liver for metabolism into several blood factors, most notably Insulin-Like-Growth-Factor (IGFI).

Studies have shown that HGH can increase exponentially following fasting – in one extreme example a man undertaking a forty day fast for religious purposes was found to have 1,250% in growth hormone by the end of the period!

But, I hear you ask, surely that means more IGFI, and didn't we learn in the science bit that insulin is the bad stuff that increases diabetes and drives fat and sugar and all of that? Isn't insulin kryptonite for the dieter? Well YES, but the key thing is in the short release time which allows the body to build resistance to the IGFI while deriving the benefits from HGH.

And those benefits are well documented – synthetic HGH is banned in athletes as a performance enhancing drug for very good reason - it increases blood glucose by driving more fat burning and greatly increases not only energy levels but also muscle mass, therefore conferring an unfair advantage.

There are no rules against naturally increasing your own HGH levels of course, and it's not just elite athletes and bodybuilders who can feel the benefits. A known (and positive) side-effect of increasing lean body mass and loss of fat is thicker and tighter skin – or in other words – ANTI-AGEING. So, you can see how there are benefits for everyone.

4.6   Suppressed Hunger

For a lot of people the biggest obstacle to taking on any dietary program (and particularly any that involve the word 'fasting'), is the thought of feeling hungry for most of the time. Nobody wants to go through their day with nagging hunger pangs following them around – hunger can decrease mood, concentration, ability to be productive, and general sense of wellbeing.

Well the good news is that IF should not make you hungry!

There is a lot of heavy science behind what makes us hungry, mostly driven by the balance of hormones including our old friends (insulin, norepinephrine and glucagon) and our bodies' response to fluctuating levels of these. Without getting further into the chemistry, it's an established fact that hunger peaks four to five hours following a meal, only for the feeling to then subside. The good news is that we can override the initial impulse to respond to our hungers pangs (as I write this my stomach is rumbling, but I don't actually feel hungry, so I'm not going to have that snack), and do this after just a couple of days of sticking to our plan.

Essentially we are learning the difference between physical hunger (with tiredness, weakness, irritability and all of that), and psychological hunger (a learned response to our hunger pangs formed out of habit). All it takes is a little perseverance, particularly in the early days. Once you've broken through the envelope, like an airliner emerging from the clouds into brilliant sunshine, you will see a better clearer world driven by the optimized processes in your body; you will have more energy, be more productive, and feel better!

4.7   Lower Cholesterol

Alongside high blood pressure and anxiety and depression, high cholesterol is possibly the most widely medicated for condition at a population level. Hundreds of millions of people worldwide are on long term medication to lower their cholesterol. At one level this makes sense – high cholesterol is a known risk factor for heart attack and stroke, and it can be regulated pharmacologically.

However, this approach is a classic example of filling the bucket and not fixing the roof. Whereas a long-term prescription for cholesterol medication may help control this risk factor, it is doing it unilaterally, with no wider benefit for the patient's health and wellbeing.

Why not assume all the benefits of lower cholesterol while also piling on the associated benefits of a better diet, lifestyle and feeling of wellbeing? And do so without the risks associated with any long-term medication – a decade or so back Pfizer pumped billions into a cholesterol management drug it called torcetrapib, designed to reduce heart attacks – in this instance by increasing the levels of "good" cholesterol (HDL) in the body. The results were staggering, staggeringly bad. Death rates of those in the study increased by a quarter - that's dozens of real people dying as they placed their trust in an experimental drug based on seemingly sound science.

Even if your medication doesn't have a weapons-grade killing capability at the population level, you still don't know what effect it is having on you and it may also provide a false sense of security that increases other risk factors in your lifestyle. The good news is that cholesterol levels can be managed, and the ratios between "good" and "bad" optimized simply by embarking on an IF programme.

4.8   Inflammation

Inflammation is defined by the Farlex medical dictionary as "A localized protective response elicited by injury or destruction of tissues, which serves to destroy, dilute, or wall off both the injurious agent and the injured tissue." Causes of inflammation include physical injury, exposure to extremes of heat or cold, infectious agents such as viruses and bacteria, and exposure to x-rays and other radioactive sources.

It is considered that almost every chronic disease is caused ultimately by INFLAMMATION, and one of the most powerful factors in increasing the likelihood of an inflammatory response to one of these triggers is - yes you've guessed it - OBESITY. Recent studies have shown that fasting induces a strong anti-inflammatory effect on the body, improving not only immune function but the nervous system in general. Once again we have a non-chemical, rapidly working and proven tool right in front of us to improve our levels of health and wellbeing.

Chapter 5: Benefits Translated

So now we have a much greater understanding of some of the benefits of intermittent fasting. Sure, some are based on stronger and more consistent science than others, but taken together a clear picture emerges of a positive impact upon body and mind. In any event, this isn't a PhD thesis, and we believe that the best way to experience the benefits is to try the plan. In this section, we look at those benefits in some more detail under the headings of our e-book and as a collective whole.

5.1   Reversing Anxiety

Anxiety affects all of us in some way and at some point in our lives, whether it's the night before our driving test, or sitting in the corridor waiting for a job interview or an important medical appointment. This form of anxiety is a natural and rational response to life events and generally has no long term ill effects, indeed the fight or flight response may be of benefit in the short term.

Problems arise when anxiety-driven responses become the normal response not only to specific and salient dangers, but to minor events that the mind blows out of proportion and fixates on, and, for a small but significant section of the population, as a continuous state of agitation and worry that cannot be switched off – what the medical profession term as Generalized Anxiety Disorder (GAD).

Anxiety issues can be plotted on a continuum from normal reactions to stressful events at one end (anxiety as a trait) to GAD at the other (anxiety as a state). But wherever you are on that graph the same set of physical symptoms are likely to accompany the mental state – including muscular tension, fatigue but inability to sleep, concentration issues and loss of appetite and libido. Given the staggering statistic that over half of GP visits in advanced countries are prompted by issues relating to anxiety, stress (and their fidgety bedfellow insomnia) it is apparent that anxiety is a MAJOR OBSTACLE to us leading not only healthy but happy, productive and fulfilled lives.

Anxiety is essentially a state of "hyperarousal", where the body remains in a revved-up state in the evening time when it should be preparing to wind down for sleep. The reason, as ever, is due to our biochemistry and is driven to a significant extent by our old friend adrenaline. In a normal state the levels of adrenaline produced in the body begin to drop in the evening, driven by the inhibitory neurotransmitter GABA (gamma aminobutyric acid) as a response to fading natural light.

Stress and anxiety counteract GABA (as does caffeine and similar stimulants), while most sleeping pills and anti-anxiety remedies are designed specifically to increase its production and counteract anxiety and insomnia. Sounds simple you might say – a straightforward pharmacological remedy to a simple problem.

Well no. Whereas a host of pharmaceutical remedies have been provided to fix this problem for going on a century now, the results have ranged from sporadic to catastrophic. From barbiturates to the range of benzodiazepine products that have flooded the market from the 1960's onwards – diazepam, Xanax, Librium –the names prompt recognition more for their infamy in public health scandals as for efficacy in doing what they were intended to.

The pharmaceutical industry response to these scandals and to the public's increasing wariness of these products was to release a new class of drug in the 1990's – the nonbenzodiazepines (see what they've done there!) which promised a more sophisticated, more targeted and safe means of treating the anxiety problem. Known colloquially as the 'Zs' (zolpidem, zaleplon and zopiclone) promised to be more effective in treating the condition without the harmful side-effects of their predecessors (which often included death, one way to overcome anxiety but not one that most of us would choose).

However, some twenty years on it is very debatable whether this has been the case, and the body of research is increasingly building a consensus of little improvement in efficacy with a list of common side-effects including daytime drowsiness, impaired coordination, dizziness, amnesia and, in the case of zopiclone, an association with cancer. And that's not even to get into the withdrawal symptoms. All in all, not exactly the prescription for a happy, energetic and productive life!

Given that we still would very much like to reduce our anxiety levels and don't have the time or the patience to wait on Big Pharma to develop the next generation to see if they're any good (definitelynotbenzodiazepines anyone?), we need to look to other remedies.

The good news is that these symptoms and the underlying anxiety itself can be tackled and overcome using IF alongside a healthy diet, good exercise regime and desire to get better, quite possibly enhanced by counseling or talking therapy.

So far we've looked at the physical advantages of IF and our 30-day plan; but what about benefits to mental health? Well the good news is that there are a range of benefits, and that IF can be deployed to wean us off antidepressants with all their side effects and dependency issues.

Low mood, which ultimately can lead to depression, is on the rise. As we have become richer we have eaten more, become less healthy and active, but our lives have become more complicated and fast-paced (think of the disappearance of the job-for-life in the past couple of generations). This perfect storm has given rise to a pandemic of depression and related mental health maladies, and the World Health Organization (WHO) predicts that by 2030 these will have become the leading source of disease burden globally. Per the definition below, disease burden calculates the overall impact of disease on a population.

Disease burden is the impact of a health problem as measured by financial cost, mortality, morbidity, or other indicators. It is often quantified in terms of quality-adjusted life years (QALYs) or disability-adjusted life years (DALYs), both of which quantify the number of years lost due to disease (YLDs)
Source: WHO

One of the leading causes of depression and low mood, as evidenced by many studies, is HIGH LEVELS OF SUGAR and INSULIN in the blood; factors which as we've already learnt here that can be mitigated by our IF program.

But it's not just the core FAT BURNING ENGINE of the IF program that will drive physiological as well as physiological benefits. A tranche of research in recent years is starting to show a clear picture of how IF can impact upon the brain directly, and in a positive manner. In rodent based tests it has been shown that IF can reduce the neurological pathology and clinical symptoms of degenerative brain diseases such as Alzheimer's and Parkinson's. Other studies have shown that calorific restriction can improve memory in the overweight and elderly and those with mild cognitive impairments, and reduce the effects of brain trauma from stroke and other cerebrovascular diseases.

At the lower end of the severity spectrum but higher end of the disease burden are depression, low mood, anxiety, ADHD and related disorders. Again, recent studies have shown clear benefits of fasting on conditions such as these.

An example is research on the Moslem month of Ramadan, a centuries old religious intermittent fast which entails restricting eating for between 11-16 hours for around a month (depending on how it falls). Large scale studies of the faithful have demonstrated reduced levels of anxiety and depression, and improved energy and mood during the holy month. This is in stark contrast to what one might think on the face of it – that a month's fast would be an ordeal typified by low energy, weakness and proneness to health problems from a weakened immune system.

As this research remains in its infancy, there no single causality factor has been identified. Theories include the increase in brain-derived neuropathic factor that arises during periods of intermittent fasting. This increases levels of naturally occurring antidepressant in the brain, stimulates new neuron growth and increases stress tolerance in the brain – essentially a mental health crash helmet.

Other theories focus on the effect of fasting on serotonin levels; as we have said more research is needed, but this is also the case with prescribed antidepressant medications, where a multi-billion-dollar industry has been built on contradictory evidence and a paradigm that dictates that they just work, somehow...

I don't know about you but given two methods of improving my mood (pharmacological and lifestyle based) that are not yet fully understood by science, I would choose the one that is guaranteed to deliver a host of other benefits without unpredictable side effects, every time.

5.2   Regaining Energy

As we've discussed above there is much about IF that seems a little counter-intuitive, and that's based upon our culturally driven perceptions of fasting as a form of suffering or even punishment. So, it is with the concept of replenishing energy by means of limiting our food intake.

Whether it's the tennis player eating a banana in her chair between games or the body builder on the high-protein diet involving all sorts of powders and shakes, the natural inclination is to believe that eating right equals high energy and high performance and so fasting equals weakness, malaise and low energy.

Well of course it's not actually that simple, even though it's incontrovertibly true that energy requires food. After all aerobic respiration operates under the formula: *Glucose + Oxygen = Energy + Carbon Dioxide + Water*, if we recall our schooldays.

As we might expect, it's the GLUCOSE element of the above equation where the crux lies. As we now know our normal (or more correctly our conditioned) eating patterns lead to ongoing dips and troughs in our blood sugar levels, and IF will move the body to a longer fed to fasted to fed cycle which allows it to switch to body fat as the primary fuel source, which will drive higher energy levels (and levels of cognitive performance).

Another major factor in this seeming paradox is the fact that metabolic rate is actually INCREASED in short-term fasting – studies have shown by as much as 10% in the first 36 to 48 hours. The reason is that adrenaline and noradrenaline levels are increased in this period, and the reason for this goes back to evolution again – to maximize survival chance humans needed to hunt or gather more food after they had eaten, and to do this requires energy.

So, the body provides this in the initial 60 hours or so after entering fasting mode, before eventually slowing down into survival and conservation mode. As none of the approaches mentioned here advocates a 60-hour plus fast, we are good on that front.

That's all well and good you may say, but if it's the case then way don't elite athletes train in a fasted state, and fast before big competitions? The answer is that MANY ACTUALLY DO and studies have shown that fasting which doesn't involve fluid restriction can lead to strength and energy levels being unaffected for up to 3.5 days of fasting (way, way beyond our method). Elite athletes will work to their own optimized programs, and many of these will involve supplements of some form, but the underlying theory still applies.

Added to all the above metabolic theory stuff is the general sense of feeling energetic that stems from feeling good about yourself, eating healthily and keeping active. We advocate that the 30-day plan is undertaken in tandem with a healthy and nutritious diet and with plenty of exercise being taken.

Once you break through the first day of hunger pangs you will start to reap the benefits of the program and feel more alert, more energetic, and more alive!

5.3   Maximizing Productivity

A standard definition of productivity is as follows:

"A measure of the efficiency of a person, machine, factory, system, etc., in converting inputs into useful outputs."

When we talk about our own productivity we mean how much we can get done in each time period based on the inputs received, and so to maximize productivity during our 30-day plan we need to be getting more done on a reduced calorific intake. To become more productive, whether our job involves looking after a baby, flying an airliner, conducting heart surgery or delivering the mail, requires a combination of mental alertness, physical energy, resistance to tiredness and lethargy, and most of all motivation to get stuff done.

Luckily, just as IF can help us avoid the route of medication to counter anxiety, so it can keep us away from the expensive supplements to be found online and in our health shops. If we briefly think back to our antelope-shaped python from above; before he struck lucky he was quite literally a different beast, alert and sinuous stalking his prey, before quickly grasping its prey, then tussling with it before asphyxiating it by constriction. In this fasted state the python is alert and productive; his metabolism optimized for the kill, as he must meet his KPI of killing again before his energy levels sap and he lapses into survival mode.

So, it is for us, in a much less dramatic and more condensed manner. Say we begin the day with a heavy breakfast – yogurt, fruit, toast, maybe even a full fry-up of sausage, bacon and eggs. Considered to be a hearty breakfast this mother-load is going to slow you down and make you feel lethargic and unproductive through the day – particularly if you follow it up with a sizeable lunch and dinner to complete your three-square meals.

You certainly shouldn't feel any hunger pangs (though the body is a demanding mistress, the more it gets the more it wants), but your waking day will be spent producing enough sugar to fuel a small army while you wearily traipse from one take to the next, wondering why you don't feel more energetic given all that nutritious food you've eaten.

Luckily IF can change all of that, and we expect your productivity to be one of the first benefits you will experience, as it can kick in almost straight away whereas the pounds and physical benefits will have a short lag. For most people, it is during the fasting period that they experience most gains, as the fast-time bodily processes fuel the benefits to your daily routine.

You are likely to notice an acute improvement in FOCUS and CONCENTRATION, and on your ability to focus on and complete analytical tasks. If your productivity is measured more by physical activity, then you that same drive and focus, and the energy benefits alluded to above, will help you do more and feel better doing it.

Although everyone is different and none of us will be impacted in precisely the same way, we are confident that, as the program continues and your body attunes to the new regime, the benefits will only increase, and your newfound energy and productivity levels will become part of who you are.

5.4   Bringing it all Together

In this section, we bring together the learning from above and present the key benefits of the 30-Day Plan to you in a single bulleted list before discussing the holistic benefits.

- Reducing Anxiety

- Lessening the state of "hyperarousal" by naturally lowering GABA (gamma aminobutyric acid)) levels in the body during the fasted period
- Removing the need for pharmacological solutions with their questionable benefits, dodgy side effects and risky withdrawal effects
- Helping on all levels of the anxiety continuum, from mild sufferers to those with gad (Generalized Anxiety Disorder)
- At a population level, an effective approach to reduce the disease burden and society's dependence on Big Pharma
- At the individual level, increasing "good" brain derived neuropathic factors stimulating neuron growth and the natural production of serotonin and other anti-depressants
- Offering clear broad-based health benefits that will increase positivity in outlook, wellbeing and build a virtuous cycle to fight anxiety and its effects
- Provide for a more stable metabolic regime to aid good sleep and lessen anxiety levels
- Reduce anxiety-driven eating disorders and free us from being imprisoned by our appetites and "comfort eating"
- Regaining Energy
  - Reprogramming the body to operate in its optimal high-fat burning state and

allowing it to derive energy from stores of body fat as opposed to spikes of glycogen feasting, thereby maximizing and regaining lost energy

- Increasing metabolic rate by up to 10% in the fasted period, driven by increased levels of adrenaline and related hormones, giving us increased energy to complete our daily tasks for up to 60 hours (just as our ancestors used it to go hunting and gathering for the next meal)
- Allowing everyone from elite athletes to the elderly and infirm to feel the benefits (though check with your physician if you have any of the risk factors identified above)
- Diverting focus from seeking out the next meal and redirecting energy to living

- Maximizing Productivity
  - Optimizing the efficiency of our conversion of food inputs to productivity outputs – allowing us to get more done
  - Avoiding the need for expensive food supplements, powders and shakes by replicating their effects from our own bodies' chemical supply
  - Increasing clarity of thought and the ability to think analytically in particular
  - Driving improved focus and concentration

- Freeing up time – 30% less meals to prepare remember!
- Above all, maximizing the motivation to do more, as you will feel healthier, more energetic and ready to get onto the next task

As we can see that is quite a list. The impressive thing about it is that all the benefits are driven from the same few internal bodily processes – it's all about the sugar and the fats – that, coupled with the right mindset will ensure we feel the benefits in short order. When we add in the specific health benefits discussed above, including reduced risk of cancer, diabetes and a host of other killers, and the fact that we can do this plan at no cost, with no impact upon our daily routine, the benefits become clear.

Chapter 6: A Sample Plan for You

Hopefully by now you are a CONVERT to IF and to the 30-Day plan we are discussing here and are ready to get thinking about your own plan. If not, that's fine, come back whenever your schedule and plans can fit it in.

Our experience is that those who find it EASIEST to adopt the plan are the following:

- Regular dieters and calorie monitoring aficionados
- Regular exercisers
- Single people or those with supportive partners / families (as skipping meals means missing social stuff)
- Flexible / home workers (again for the social aspect but also because initial transition is easier managed)

Whereas the following may find it more difficult:

- Married with children (particularly young children)
- Client facing jobs
- Diet and exercise rookies
- The more elderly (set in routine)

If you fall into the latter group, or if you're just not ready to take the plunge for whatever reason, then take some baby steps first; skip the odd meal, disobey those routine-driven hunger pangs every now and again. We'll hopefully see you again when you're good and ready – IF works best when it's part of your regular routine; nobody is making you do it and the last it's meant to be is a source of self-imposed stress.

If you are ready to go, then great, we'll next move into a brief example of what your plan may look like – start to put this theory into practice.

Remember this isn't a prescription – feel free to tweak so it works for your schedule, lifestyle and what you like to eat – remember it's fasting for benefit, not punishment or penance!

6.1   Defining your Goals

Before you start you need what it is you want to achieve. And that's going to vary a lot depending on whether you're a sixty-something, a little overweight and most concerned about diabetes and high cholesterol, or a fit and healthy twenty-something looking to optimize that already good BMI index and maximize your energy and productivity.

Most of us will have heard about the SMART goals mnemonic (easy to write, hard to say!) from school, business or general management-speak, but it's a pretty good way to set goals, so we'll use the approach here:

- SPECIFIC -Per above, target your ONE AREA for improvement
- MEASUREABLE - How are you going to measure success?
- ACHIEVEABLE - e.g. not losing 25% of your body weight in a month
- RESPONSIBLE - Easy peasy, it's your goal, you alone are responsible
- TIME RELATED - 30 days for this plan, but you may go more long term

Take some time on this exercise and ensure you've got the goal right, because you may a few competing priorities but you want to make sure you target the plan to what's best for you.

6.2   Set your Goal Metrics

Put some thought into what metrics you will use to see if your plan is working for you and if you are on target to meet your goal. As we mentioned above, body weight is an obvious metric, but equally body mass index could be your think, or cholesterol level, or if you're more sophisticated and prepared to have some diagnostics run, any blood marker you care to choose.

Alternatively, you could go down a different route and run some metrics on your own fitness through the plan – e.g. your time for 100-meter sprint or how much you can bench-press. Or you can set less strenuous sounding goals connected with your general wellbeing – estimated hours sleep per night, feeling of energy or motivation (though use your own quantitative scale if you can).

As you can see the possibilities are endless, and you should have some fun coming up with the best plan for you.

6.3   Set your Baseline Metrics

There's nothing to start you jumping right into the plan, but if you have some time it's a good idea to baseline your metrics before you start. This is particularly for those on the higher performance end of the scale – you'll know that your factors, whether it's your body weight, running speed or your blood markers will vary depending on when collecting, so it's a good idea to have some average values. If you think this is overkill for your requirements that's fine, on to the next section it is!

6.4   Look at your Diet

As with your measurement variables, it's a good idea to take a step back and look at your diet before you start the plan. Whether you eat consistently every week or whether your diet varies depending on where you are, who you are with or any other factors, it's a good idea to get a view on what is standard for you.

If you are approaching this in a relatively casual manner – you eat pretty much what you eat and will continue to do so over the 30 days, then that is no problem whatsoever. We're not looking for everyone to log all their calories, we just want you to have an idea – the degree of accuracy dependent on your goals and priorities – of what you have consumed through the trial and that inconsistency isn't going to skew your numbers at the end of it.

Another reason for doing this is if you believe your diet as it is now being deficient or particularly unhealthy. If you have any doubts in this regard, then discuss with your physician and a dietician before you set out. Ultimately you will be consuming on average 30% of your normal caloric intake and you need to be confident that this will not cause any issues.

Please see statement above if you have any other doubts as to your suitability on general grounds of health.

6.5   Finalize your Plan

The core plan proposed here is based around Eat-Stop-Eat, with fasting for two 24 hour days each week (supper to supper).

6.5.1 Timing

We are proposing the above schedule (though as said you can do a lesser or greater level of fasting as you wish (but don't go too high on the fasting days!). In terms of breaking this out into a 30-Day plan we provide a simple table below, for an indicative 30 day month starting on a Monday. We're going to fast on a Sunday and a Wednesday (we'll ease ourselves in).

	Monday	Tuesday	Wednesday	Thursday	Friday	Saturday	Sunday
Week 1	Normal intake	Normal intake	All-day fast	Normal intake	Normal intake	Normal intake	All-day fast
Week 2	Normal intake	Normal intake	All-day fast	Normal intake	Normal intake	Normal intake	All-day fast
Week 3	Normal intake	Normal intake	All-day fast	Normal intake	Normal intake	Normal intake	All-day fast
Week 4	Normal intake	Normal intake	All-day fast	Normal intake	Normal intake	Normal intake	All-day fast
Week 5	Normal intake	Normal intake					

6.5.2 Calendaring your Plan

This is our basic plan. It's simple but also quite intensive particularly for a first-time follower. Think about your requirements before embarking on it: remember we can easily switch from Eat-Stop-Eat to a 5:2 diet – where we allow ourselves 25% of our normal intake on fasting days, in which case our table will look like the below.

Remember the SMART approach and your goals before committing to your plan.

	Monday	Tuesday	Wednesday	Thursday	Friday	Saturday	Sunday
Week 1	normal intake	normal intake	25% normal intake	normal intake	norma l	normal intake	25%
Week 2	normal intake	normal intake	25% normal intake	normal intake	norma l	normal intake	25%
Week 3	normal intake	normal intake	25% normal intake	normal intake	norma l	normal intake	25%
Week 4	normal intake	normal intake	25% normal intake	normal intake	norma l	normal intake	25%
Week 5	normal intake	normal intake					

6.5.3 Monitoring Intake and Exercise

Again, following SMART, we can build further metrics and variables into our planner. For example, you may wish to log the calorific content of your meals in the plan, or to add a section to log the level of exercise you have undertaken each day. As we've said before, how simple or how complex you wish to make your study is entirely up to you.

Whichever variant of the plan you decide to follow, or if you opt for an amalgam or an IF schedule of your own devising, ensure to follow it as closely as you can, but also ensure that you are making it work for you.

Don't be afraid to chop and change your approach if you are experiencing any negatives, or if it's not fitting with your lifestyle. Intermittent Fasting is meant to be fun, as well as your ticket to a happier, less anxious and more energetic and productive life.

We're confident that once you try it and find the right fit for you, you won't want to return to your three-square meal eating habits of old.

Don't take our word for it, get out there and start thinking about your plan today!

Conclusion

Thank you again for downloading this book!

I hope this book could help you to reverse anxiety, regain your energy and increase your productivity.

The next step is get results by taking MAXIMUM ACTION in Intermittent Fasting.

Finally, if you enjoyed this book, then I'd like to ask you for a favour, would you be kind enough to leave a review for this book on Amazon? It'd be greatly appreciated!

Click here to leave a review for this book on Amazon!

Thank you and good luck!

Printed in Great Britain
by Amazon